49 Juicing Solutions to Reduce Muscle Cramps:

Eliminate Painful Muscle Cramps Using Natures Ingredients

By

Joe Correa CSN

COPYRIGHT

ACKNOWLEDGEMENTS

This book is dedicated to my friends and family that have had mild or serious illnesses so that you may find a solution and make the necessary changes in your life.

49 Juicing Solutions to Reduce Muscle Cramps:

Eliminate Painful Muscle Cramps Using Natures Ingredients

By

Joe Correa CSN

CONTENTS

ABOUT THE AUTHOR

After years of Research, I honestly believe in the positive effects that proper nutrition can have over the body and mind. My knowledge and experience has helped me live healthier throughout the years and which I have shared with family and friends. The more you know about eating and drinking healthier, the sooner you will want to change your life and eating habits.

Nutrition is a key part in the process of being healthy and living longer so get started today. The first step is the most important and the most significant.

INTRODUCTION

49 Juicing Solutions to Reduce Muscle Cramps: Eliminate Painful Muscle Cramps Using Natures Ingredients

By Joe Correa CSN

The involuntary and rather painful condition of a contracted muscle that doesn't relax is something we have all experienced at least once in our life. Usually, the condition is quite harmless and it only lasts for a couple of minutes during which the person is unable to use the affected muscle.

Muscle cramps are often caused by difficult exercises, hard physical labor, dehydration, or use of certain medications. They can occur in almost every muscle in the body, especially in the leg and feet muscles. As I said earlier, most of the time muscle cramps are harmless, however, sometimes they can be related to some more serious medical condition like:

- Inadequate blood supply due to narrowed arteries causes muscle cramps during exercise.
- Nerve compression in the spine is related to muscle cramps while walking,

- Lack of minerals like potassium, calcium, or magnesium in your body can also lead to muscle cramps.

In some cases, it is highly recommended to visit a doctor, especially if you feel severe pain, muscle weakness, leg swelling, rashes or any other skin changes. Also, if you suffer from frequent muscle cramps that don't improve over time, medical attention is necessary.

Although muscle cramps can happen to everyone for various reasons, there are some risk factors that increase this painful condition. These factors include age, different medical conditions, and dehydration. Older people who lose their muscle mass are frequently affected by muscle cramps, even during some relatively easy physical activities. Pregnant women and people suffering from diabetes, thyroid or liver disorders also experience frequent and harmless muscle cramps. Finally, dehydration during long physical activities (especially in hot weather) is often the cause of muscle cramps.

There are a couple of simple steps that will help prevent muscle cramps. As mentioned above, muscle cramps are often related to dehydration which means that keeping your body fully hydrated all the time is crucial to avoid this painful condition. Drinking plenty of fresh juices will have an amazing effect on your entire body, including muscle cramps.

This collection of muscle cramp reducing juice recipes will keep your body hydrated all the time and provide a rich amount of different nutrients you need on a daily basis.

Take a couple of minutes every day to prepare one of these delicious recipes and forget about having muscle cramps once and for all.

COMMITMENT

In order to improve my condition, I *(your name)*, commit to eating more of these foods on a daily basis and to exercise at least 30 minutes daily:

- Berries (especially blueberries), peaches, cherries, apples, apricots, oranges, lemon juice, grapefruit, tangerines, mandarins, pears, etc.
- Broccoli, spinach, collard greens, sweet potatoes, avocado, artichoke, baby corn, carrots, celery, cauliflower, onions, etc.
- Whole grains, steel-cut oats, oatmeal, quinoa, barley, etc.
- Black beans, red bean beans, garbanzo beans, lentils, etc.
- Nuts and seeds including: walnuts, cashews, flaxseeds, sesame seeds, etc.
- Fish
- 8 – 10 glasses of water

Sign here

X_____

49 JUICING SOLUTIONS TO REDUCE MUSCLE CRAMPS

1. Watermelon Banana Juice

Ingredients:

1 cup of watermelon, diced

1 large banana, chunked

1 medium-sized wedge of honeydew melon

1 small ginger knob, peeled and chopped

1 medium-sized carrot, sliced

Preparation:

Cut the top of the watermelon. Cut lengthwise in half and then cut one large wedge. Peel it and cut into small cubes. Remove the seeds and fill the measuring cup. Wrap the rest in a plastic foil and refrigerate for later.

Peel the banana and cut into chunks. Set aside.

Cut the honeydew melon in half. Cut one large wedge and peel the peel it. Cut into small pieces and set aside. Wrap the rest of the melon in a plastic foil and refrigerate.

Peel the ginger and cut into small pieces. Set aside.

Wash and peel the carrot. Cut into thin slices and set aside.

Now, combine watermelon, banana, honeydew melon, ginger, and carrot in a juicer. Process until juiced.

Transfer to a serving glass and add some crushed ice before serving.

Enjoy!

Nutrition information per serving: Kcal: 230, Protein: 4.3g, Carbs: 75.8g, Fats: 1.2g

2. Cucumber Pomegranate Juice

Ingredients:

1 large orange, peeled

1 large cucumber, sliced

1 cup of pomegranate seeds

1 cup of purple cabbage, torn

1 cup of sweet potatoes, cubed

4 oz of water

Preparation:

Wash the cucumber and cut into thick slices. Set aside.

Cut the top of the pomegranate fruit using a sharp knife. Slice down to each of the white membranes inside of the fruit. Pop the seeds into a measuring cup and set aside.

Peel the orange and divide into wedges. Set aside.

Wash the cabbage thoroughly under cold running water. Drain and torn with hands. Set aside.

Peel the sweet potato and cut into cubes. Fill the measuring cup and reserve the rest for another juice. Set aside.

Now, combine orange, pomegranate seeds, purple cabbage, sweet potatoes, and cucumber in a juicer and process until juiced.

Transfer to serving glasses and stir in the water. Add some ice cubes and serve immediately.

Enjoy!

Nutritional information per serving: Kcal: 251, Protein: 6.8g, Carbs: 73.1g, Fats: 1.5g

3.   Squash Raspberry Juice

Ingredients:

1 cup butternut squash, chopped

1 cup raspberries

2 cups cantaloupe, chopped

1 large apricot, chopped

1 large kiwi, peeled

Preparation:

Peel the butternut squash and cut in half. Scoop out the seeds using a spoon. Cut into small chunks and set aside. Reserve the rest for another juice.

Rinse the raspberries under cold running water using a large colander. Set aside.

Cut the cantaloupe in half. Scoop out the seeds and flesh. Cut two wedges and peel them. Chop into chunks and set aside. Reserve the rest of the cantaloupe in a refrigerator.

Wash the apricot and cut in half. Remove the pit and cut into chunks. Set aside.

Peel the kiwi and cut lengthwise in half. Set aside.

Now, combine squash, raspberries, cantaloupe, apricots, and kiwi in a juicer.

Transfer to serving glasses and add some ice before serving.

Enjoy!

Nutritional information per serving: Kcal: 193, Protein: 6.6g, Carbs: 59.1g, Fats: 2.3g

4. Banana Apple Juice

Ingredients:

1 large banana, sliced

1 small Golden Delicious apple, cored

2 cups blueberries

1 large cucumber, sliced

3 oz water

Preparation:

Peel the banana and cut into small chunks. Set aside.

Wash the apple and remove the core. Cut into bite-sized pieces and set aside.

Place the blueberries in a colander and wash under cold running water. Drain and set aside.

Wash the cucumber and cut into thick slices. Set aside.

Now, process banana, apple, blueberries, and cucumber in a juicer. Transfer to serving glasses and add some ice before serving.

Enjoy!

Nutritional information per serving: Kcal: 348, Protein: 6g, Carbs: 102g, Fats: 1.9g

5.   Watermelon Maple Juice

Ingredients:

1 cup of watermelon, diced

1 tbsp of maple syrup

1 cup plums, pitted and halved

1 large Granny Smith apple, cored

3 oz of water

Preparation:

Cut the watermelon lengthwise. For one cup, you will need about 1 large wedge. Peel and cut into chunks. Remove the seeds and set aside. Reserve the rest of the melon for some other juices.

Wash the plums and cut into halves. Remove the pits and fill the measuring cup. Set aside.

Wash the apple and remove the core. Cut into bite-sized pieces and set aside.

Now, combine watermelon, plums, and apple in a juicer. Process until juiced.

Transfer to serving glasses and stir in the maple syrup and water. Optionally, add some ice or refrigerate before serving.

Enjoy!

Nutritional information per serving: Kcal: 335, Protein: 4.3g, Carbs: 96.8g, Fats: 1.6g

6.   Strawberry Apple Juice

Ingredients:

1 cup strawberries, chopped

1 large Fuji apple, chopped

1 cup pomegranate seeds

1 large orange, peeled

1 cup fresh spinach

2 oz water

Preparation:

Rinse the strawberries under running water and remove the stems. Chop into small pieces and fill the measuring cup. Set aside.

Wash the apple and remove the core. Cut into bite-sized pieces and set aside.

Cut the top of the pomegranate fruit using a sharp knife. Slice down to each of the white membranes inside of the fruit. Pop the seeds into a medium bowl.

Rinse the spinach thoroughly and torn into small pieces. Set aside.

Peel the orange and divide into wedges. Set aside.

Now, process strawberries, apple, pomegranate seeds, spinach, and orange in a juicer. Transfer to serving glasses and stir in the water.

Refrigerate for 10 minutes before serving.

Nutritional information per serving: Kcal: 266, Protein: 6.1g, Carbs: 80.8g, Fats: 2.2g

7.   Mango Plum Juice

Ingredients:

1 cup mango, chopped

3 large plums, pitted

1 large grapefruit, peeled

1 medium-sized green apple, cored

2 oz coconut water

2 tbsp fresh mint, finely chopped

Preparation:

Peel the mango and cut into chunks. Fill the measuring cup and refrigerate the rest for some other juice. Set aside.

Wash the plums and cut in half. Remove the pits and chop into small pieces. Set aside.

Peel the grapefruit and divide into wedges. Cut each wedge in half and set aside.

Wash the apple and remove the core. Cut into bite-sized pieces and set aside.

Now, combine mango, plums, grapefruit, and apple in a juicer. Process until juiced. Transfer to serving glasses and stir in the coconut water.

Add a few ice cubes and garnish with mint.

Serve immediately.

Nutritional information per serving: Kcal: 211, Protein: 9.3g, Carbs: 59.3g, Fats: 1.5g

8.   Melon Agave Juice

Ingredients:

1 cup watermelon, seeded

1 cup honeydew melon, chopped

1 cup pomegranate seeds

1 cup beets, trimmed

2 medium-sized radishes, chopped

1 tbsp agave nectar

Preparation:

Cut the watermelon lengthwise. For one cup, you will need about 1 large wedge. Peel and cut into chunks. Remove the seeds and set aside. Reserve the rest of the melon for some other juices.

Cut the honeydew melon lengthwise in half. Scoop out the seeds using a spoon. Cut into large wedges and peel them. Now, cut into small chunks and place in a bowl. Set aside.

Wash the beets and radishes and trim off the green parts. Chop into small pieces and set aside.

Cut the top of the pomegranate fruit using a sharp knife. Slice down to each of the white membranes inside of the fruit. Pop the seeds into a measuring cup and set aside.

Now, combine watermelon, honeydew melon, beets, and pomegranate seeds in a juicer. Process until juiced.

Transfer to serving glasses and stir in the agave nectar.

Add some ice and serve.

Nutrition information per serving: Kcal: 167, Protein: 13.1g, Carbs: 45.9g, Fats: 1.5g

9.   Cherry Lime Juice

Ingredients:

1 cup honeydew melon, chopped

1 cup sour cherries

1 large lime, peeled

1 large orange, peeled

1 tbsp honey

2 oz coconut water

Preparation:

Rinse the cherries using a colander and cut in half. Remove the pits and set aside.

Peel the lime and cut lengthwise in half. Set aside.

Cut the honeydew melon lengthwise in half. Scoop out the seeds using a spoon. Cut the large wedges and peel them. Cut into small chunks and place in a bowl. Wrap the rest of the melon in a plastic foil and refrigerate.

Peel the orange and divide into wedges. Set aside.

Now, combine cherries, lime, melon, and orange in a juicer. Transfer to serving glasses and stir in the honey and coconut water.

Add some ice and serve immediately.

Nutritional information per serving: Kcal: 276, Protein: 4.2g, Carbs: 78.9g, Fats: 0.7g

10.   Lemon Lime Juice

Ingredients:

2 large lemons, peeled

2 large limes, peeled

3 large oranges, peeled

¼ tsp ginger powder

1 tbsp maple syrup

2 oz water

Preparation:

Peel the lemons and limes and cut lengthwise in half. Set aside.

Peel the oranges and divide into wedges. Cut each wedge in half and set aside.

Now, combine oranges, lemons, and limes in a juicer.

Transfer to serving glasses and stir in the cinnamon, maple syrup, and water.

Add few ice cubes and serve immediately.

Nutrition information per serving: Kcal: 246, Protein: 6.8g, Carbs: 83.1g, Fats: 1.1g

11.   Orange Grape Juice

Ingredients:

1 large blood orange, peeled

1 cup black grapes

1 cup asparagus, trimmed

1 large lemon, peeled

1 large lime, peeled

3 oz water

Preparation:

Peel the orange and divide into wedges. Set aside.

Wash the green grapes under cold running water. Drain water and set aside.

Wash the asparagus and trim off the woody ends. Cut into 1-inch pieces and set aside.

Peel the lemon and lime and cut lengthwise in half. Set aside.

Now, combine orange, grapes, asparagus, lemon, and lime in a juicer. Process until juiced.

Transfer to serving glasses and stir in the water. Add some ice and serve immediately.

Enjoy!

Nutritional information per serving: Kcal: 361, Protein: 5.1g, Carbs: 109g, Fats: 1.5g

12. Honeydew Cantaloupe Juice

Ingredients:

1 large banana, chopped

¼ tsp cinnamon, ground

1 cup honeydew melon, cubed

1 cup cantaloupe, diced

Preparation:

Peel the banana and cut into small pieces. Set aside.

Cut the melon lengthwise in half. For one cup, cut one large wedge. Peel and chop into small cubes. Remove the seeds and fill the measuring cup. Reserve the rest in the refrigerator.

Cut the cantaloupe in half and scoop out the seeds. Cut and peel two medium wedges. Fill the measuring cup and reserve the rest for later.

Now, combine banana, melon, and cantaloupe in a juicer and process until juiced. Transfer to a serving glass and stir in the cinnamon. Refrigerate for 5 minutes before serving.

Enjoy!

Nutrition information per serving: Kcal: 171, Protein: 3.4g, Carbs: 47.3g, Fats: 0.8g

13.　Watermelon Banana Juice

Ingredients:

1 cup watermelon, diced

1 medium-sized banana, sliced

1 cup celery, chopped

¼ tsp ginger, ground

2 oz water

Preparation:

Cut the watermelon in half. Cut and peel one large wedge. Dice into small pieces and remove the seeds. Fill the measuring cup and wrap the rest of the melon in a plastic foil. Refrigerate for later.

Peel the banana and cut into slices. Set aside.

Wash the celery and cut into bite-sized pieces. Fill the measuring cup and reserve the rest for later.

Now, combine watermelon, banana, and celery in a juicer and process until juiced. Transfer to a serving glass and stir in the water and ginger.

Add some ice and serve immediately.

Enjoy!

Nutrition information per serving: Kcal: 147, Protein: 2.9g, Carbs: 41.4g, Fats: 0.8g

14.   Cinnamon Peach Juice

Ingredients:

3 large peaches, pitted and chopped

1 cup pineapple, peeled and chunked

¼ tsp cinnamon, ground

½ cup cantaloupe, chopped

1 oz water

Preparation:

Wash the peaches and cut in half. Remove the pits and cut into bite-sized pieces. Set aside.

Cut the top of the pineapple and peel it using a sharp paring knife. Peel it all and cut into small pieces. Fill the measuring cup and set aside.

Cut the cantaloupe in half and scoop out the seeds. Cut and peel two medium wedges. Fill the measuring cup and reserve the rest for later.

Now, combine peaches, cantaloupe, and pineapple in a juicer and process until juiced. Transfer to a serving glass and stir in the cinnamon.

Refrigerate for 10 minutes before serving.

Nutrition information per serving: Kcal: 237, Protein: 5.4g, Carbs: 69.1g, Fats: 5.4g

15.   Watermelon Swiss Chard Juice

Ingredients:

1 cup watermelon, diced

2 cups Swiss chard, chopped

1 cup pineapple, chunked

¼ tsp ginger, ground

Preparation:

Cut the top of the watermelon. Cut lengthwise in half and then cut one large wedge. Peel it and cut into small cubes. Remove the seeds and fill the measuring cup. Wrap the rest in a plastic foil and refrigerate for later.

Rinse the Swiss chard thoroughly under cold running water. Slightly drain and chop into small pieces. Set aside.

Cut the top of the pineapple and peel it using a sharp paring knife. Peel it all and cut into small pieces. Fill the measuring cup and set aside.

Now, combine watermelon, Swiss chard, and pineapple in a juicer. Process until juiced. Transfer to a serving glass and stir in the ginger.

Add some ice and serve immediately.

Enjoy!

Nutrition information per serving: Kcal: 127, Protein: 3.1g, Carbs: 35.8g, Fats: 0.6g

16.   Mint Apple Juice

Ingredients:

1 cup fresh mint, chopped

1 small Granny Smith's apple, cored

1 large guava, chopped

2 oz water

Preparation:

Wash the mint thoroughly under cold running water. Chop into small pieces and set aside.

Wash the apple and cut in half. Remove the core and cut into bite-sized pieces. Set aside.

Peel the guava and cut lengthwise in half. Scoop out the seeds and chop into small pieces. Set aside.

Now, combine mint, apple, and guava in a juicer and process until juiced. Transfer to a serving glass and stir in the water.

Refrigerate for 5 minutes before serving.

Enjoy!

Nutrition information per serving: Kcal: 288, Protein: 4.4g, Carbs: 91.7g, Fats: 1.6g

17.   Apple Pomegranate Juice

Ingredients:

1 large Granny Smith's apple, chopped

1 cup of pomegranate seeds

1 large peach, pitted and halved

3 oz of water

1 tbsp agave nectar

Preparation:

Wash the apple and cut in half. Remove the core and cut into bite-sized pieces. Set aside.

Cut the top of the pomegranate fruit using a sharp knife. Slice down to each of the white membranes inside of the fruit. Pop the seeds into measuring cup and set aside.

Wash the peach and cut in half. Remove the pit and cut into small pieces. Set aside.

Now, combine apple, pomegranate seeds, and peach in a juicer and process until juiced.

Transfer to serving glasses and stir in the water and agave nectar.

Add some ice and serve!

Nutrition information per serving: Kcal: 212, Protein: 3.9g, Carbs: 61g, Fats: 1.8g

18.   Cucumber Mango Juice

Ingredients:

1 cup blueberries

1 cup cucumber, sliced

1 cup mango, chunked

1 medium-sized green apple, cored

2 oz water

Preparation:

Peel the cucumber and cut into slices. Fill the measuring cup and reserve the rest for later.

Wash the mango and cut into chunks. Fill the measuring cup and reserve the rest for some other juice. Set aside.

Rinse the blueberries under cold running water using a colander. Drain and set aside.

Wash the apple and remove the core. Cut into bite-sized pieces and set aside.

Now, combine cucumber, mango, blueberries, and apple in a juicer. Process until juiced.

Transfer to a serving glass and stir in the water. Add some ice before serving and enjoy!

Nutrition information per serving: Kcal: 178, Protein: 5.8g, Carbs: 61.5g, Fats: 1.1g

19.   Zucchini Grape Juice

Ingredients:

1 small zucchini, chopped

1 cup black grapes

1 medium-sized pear, chopped

¼ tsp cinnamon, ground

2 oz water

Preparation:

Peel the zucchini and cut into bite-sized cubes. Set aside.

Wash the grapes and fill the measuring cup. Set aside.

Wash the pear and cut in half. Remove the core and cut into small pieces. Set aside.

Now, combine zucchini, grapes, and pear in a juicer. Process until juiced. Transfer to a serving glass and stir in the cinnamon and water.

Add some crushed ice and serve immediately.

Enjoy!

Nutrition information per serving: Kcal: 153, Protein: 2.6 g, Carbs: 46.6g, Fats: 0.9g

20.   Apple Cucumber Juice

Ingredients:

1 large Granny Smith's apple, chopped

1 large cucumber, sliced

2 large honeydew melon wedges

2 oz of water

Preparation:

Wash and peel the apple. Cut in half and remove the core. Cut into bite-sized pieces and set aside.

Peel the cucumber. Cut into thin slices and set aside.

Cut the honeydew melon lengthwise in half. Scoop out the seeds using a spoon. Cut two large wedges and peel them. Cut into small chunks and fill the measuring cup. Wrap the rest of the melon in a plastic foil and refrigerate.

Now, combine apple, cucumber, and honeydew melon in a juicer. Process until juiced. Transfer to serving glasses and stir in the water.

Add some ice before serving and enjoy!

Nutrition information per serving: Kcal: 241, Protein: 4.6g, Carbs: 68.1g, Fats: 1.2g

21.   Peach Lemon Juice

Ingredients:

1 large peach, pitted and halved

1 large lemon, peeled

1 large orange, peeled

1 medium-sized cucumber, sliced

1 cup pomegranate seeds

2 oz water

1 tbsp of maple syrup

Preparation:

Wash the peach and cut in half. Remove the pit and cut into small pieces. Set aside.

Peel the lemon and cut lengthwise in half. Set aside.

Peel the orange and divide into wedges. Set aside.

Wash the cucumber and cut into thin slices. Set aside.

Cut the top of the pomegranate fruit using a sharp knife. Slice down to each of the white membranes inside of the fruit. Pop the seeds into measuring cup and set aside.

Now, combine peach, lemon, orange, cucumber, and pomegranate seeds in a juicer. Process until juiced.

Transfer to serving glasses and stir in the water and maple syrup.

Refrigerate for 5 minutes before serving.

Nutrition information per serving: Kcal: 265, Protein: 5.6g, Carbs: 63.7g, Fats: 1.8g

22.   Radish Apple Juice

Ingredients:

1 cup radishes, chopped

1 medium-sized apple, peeled and wedged

1 large orange, peeled

1 cup Romain lettuce, torn

1 cup watercress, torn

1 tbsp honey

Preparation:

Wash the radishes and trim off the green parts. Cut into small pieces and fill the measuring cup. Set aside.

Wash the apple and cut in half. Remove the core and chop into small pieces. Set aside.

Peel the orange and divide into wedges. Set aside.

Rinse the lettuce and watercress using a large colander. Drain and torn with hands.

Now, combine radishes, apple, orange, lettuce, and watercress in a juicer. Process until juiced.

Transfer to serving glasses and add some ice before serving.

Enjoy!

Nutrition information per serving: Kcal: 150, Protein: 7.3g, Carbs: 53.4g, Fats: 0.8g

23.   Apple Beet Juice

Ingredients:

1 large Honeycrisp apple, cored

2 medium-sized beets, trimmed

1 large cucumber, sliced

1 whole lime, peeled

¼ tsp ginger powder

Preparation:

Wash the apple and remove the core. Cut into bite-sized pieces and set aside.

Wash the beets and trim off the green ends. Save it for another juice. Cut the beet into small pieces. Set aside.

Wash the cucumber and cut it into thick slices. Set aside.

Peel the lime and cut into quarters. Set aside.

Now, process apple, beets, cucumber, and lime in a juicer. Transfer to serving glasses and add some ice before serving.

Enjoy!

Nutrition information per serving: Kcal: 109, Protein: 2.8g, Carbs: 33.6g, Fats: 0.7g

24. Apricot Mango Juice

Ingredients:

1 cup apricots, sliced

1 cup mango, chopped

½ cup coconut water

1 tbsp maple syrup

Preparation:

Wash the apricots and cut in half. Remove the pits and chop into small pieces. Set aside.

Peel the mango and cut into small chunks. Fill the measuring cup and rserve the rest in the refrigerator.

Now, combine apricots, mango, and coconut water in a juicer. Process until juiced.

Transfer to serving glasses and stir in the maple syrup.

Add few ice cubes and serve immediately.

Nutrition information per serving: Kcal: 155, Protein: 3.6g, Carbs: 43g, Fats: 1.2g

25.   Basil Raspberry Juice

Ingredients:

1 cup fresh basil, torn

2 cups raspberries

1 cup beets, chopped

1 large Granny Smith's apple, cored

1 whole lemon, peeled

3 oz water

Preparation:

Wash the basil thoroughly under cold running water and torn with hands. Set aside.

Wash the raspberries under cold running water using a colander. Drain and set aside.

Wash the beets and trim off the green ends. Cut into small pieces and fill the measuring cup. Reserve the greens for some other juice.

Wash the apple and cut in half. Remove the core and cut into bite-sized pieces. Set aside.

Peel the lemon and cut lengthwise in half. Set aside.

Now, combine basil, raspberries, beets, apple, and lemon in a juicer. Process until well juiced.

Stir in the water and refrigerate for 10-15 minutes before serving.

Enjoy!

Nutrition information per serving: Kcal: 218, Protein: 7.5g, Carbs: 76.4g, Fats: 2.5g

26.   Strawberry Grapefruit Juice

Ingredients:

2 large strawberries, chopped

2 large grapefruits, peeled

1 large Red Delicious apple, cored

1 small ginger knob, peeled

2 oz coconut water

Preparation:

Rinse the strawberries using a colander. Remove the green stems and cut into small pieces. Set aside.

Peel the grapefruits and divide into wedges. Cut each wedge in half and set aside.

Wash the apple and cut in half. Remove the core and cut into bite-sized pieces. Set aside.

Peel the ginger knob and set aside.

Now, combine strawberries, grapefruit, apple, and ginger in a juicer. Process until well juiced.

Transfer to serving glasses and stir in the coconut water. Refrigerate for 5 minutes before serving.

Enjoy!

Nutrition information per serving: Kcal: 302, Protein: 4.8g, Carbs: 86.3g, Fats: 1.7g

27.   Apricot Raspberry Juice

Ingredients:

3 whole apricots, pitted

1 cup fresh blackberries

1 cup fresh raspberries

1 large Fuji apple, cored

3 large carrots, peeled and sliced

Preparation:

Combine blackberries and raspberries in a colander. Rinse well under cold running water and slightly drain. Set aside.

Wash the apricots and cut in half. Remove the pits and cut into bite-sized pieces. Set aside.

Wash the apple and cut in half. Remove the core and cut into small pieces.

Wash and peel the carrots. Cut into thin slices and set aside.

Now, combine apricots, raspberries, blackberries, apple, and carrots in a juicer. Process until well juiced and transfer to serving glasses. Stir in the water and refrigerate for 5 minutes before serving.

Enjoy!

Nutrition information per serving: Kcal: 301, Protein: 7.6g, Carbs: 97.4g, Fats: 2.9g

28.   Mint Strawberry Juice

Ingredients:

1 cup fresh mint, chopped

1 cup strawberries, chopped

1 cup avocado, pitted

1 large Honeycrisp apple, cored and chopped

1 large lemon, peeled

1 large cucumber, sliced

Preparation:

Wash the mint thoroughly and torn with hands. Set aside.

Wash the strawberries and cut into small pieces. Set aside.

Peel the avocado and cut lengthwise in half. Remove the pit and cut into chunks and fill the measuring cup. Reserve the rest for later.

Wash the apple and cut in half. Remove the core and cut into bite-sized pieces. Set aside.

Peel the lemon and cut lengthwise in half. Set aside.

Peel the cucumber and cut into thin slices. Set aside.

Now, combine mint, strawberries, avocado, lemon, and cucumber in a juicer. Process until juiced. Transfer to serving glasses and stir in the water.

Add some ice before serving.

Nutrition information per serving: Kcal: 376, Protein: 8.1g, Carbs: 67.8g, Fats: 23.3g

29.   Orange Cranberry Juice

Ingredients:

1 large orange, peeled

1 cup fresh cranberries

1 cup fresh strawberries

2 oz coconut water

Preparation:

Combine cranberries and strawberries in a colander. Rinse under cold running water. Drain and set aside.

Peel the orange and divide into wedges. Cut each wedge in half and set aside.

Combine cranberries, strawberries, and orange in a juicer. Process until juiced.

Transfer to serving glasses and stir in the coconut water.

Add some ice and serve immediately.

Nutrition information per serving: Kcal: 137, Protein: 3.2g, Carbs: 46.6g, Fats: 0.8g

30.   Grape Beet Juice

Ingredients:

1 cup black grapes

1 cup beets, trimmed and sliced

1 large blood orange, peeled

1 whole apricot, pitted

1 tbsp coconut water

Preparation:

Rinse the grapes and remove the stems. Set aside.

Wash the beets and trim off the green parts. Cut into thin slices and fill the measuring cup. Reserve the rest for later.

Peel the orange and divide into wedges. Cut each wedge in half and set aside.

Wash the apricot and cut lengthwise in half. Remove the pit and cut into small pieces. Set aside.

Now, combine grapes, beets, orange, and apricots in a juicer and process until well juiced. Transfer to a serving glass and stir in the coconut water.

Add some ice and serve immediately.

Nutrition information per serving: Kcal: 184, Protein: 4.9g, Carbs: 54.3g, Fats: 0.9g

31.   Banana Apricot Juice

Ingredients:

1 medium-sized banana, sliced

3 whole apricots, chopped

1 medium-sized celery stalk, chopped

1 small Fuji apple, chopped

1 tsp maple syrup

1 oz water

Preparation:

Peel the banana and cut into small chunks. Set aside.

Rinse the apricots and cut in half. Remove the pits and cut into bite-sized pieces. Set aside.

Rinse the celery stalk and cut into bite-sized pieces. Set aside.

Wash the apple and cut in half. Remove the core and cut into bite-sized pieces. Set aside.

Now, combine banana, apricots, celery, and apple in a juicer and process until juiced. Transfer to a serving glass and stir in the maple syrup and add few ice cubes.

Serve immediately.

Nutrition information per serving: Kcal: 185, Protein: 3.6g, Carbs: 68.8g, Fats: 1.6g

32.   Beet Carrot Juice

Ingredients:

1 cup beets, trimmed

1 large carrot, sliced

1 cup avocado, chopped

1 small ginger knob, 1-inch thick

2 oz water

Preparation:

Trim off the green parts of the beets. Peel and cut into thin slices. Fill the measuring cup and reserve the remaining beet in the refrigerator.

Wash and peel the carrot. Cut into bite-sized pieces and set aside.

Peel the avocado and cut lengthwise in half. Remove the pit and cut into bite-sized pieces. Fill the measuring cup and reserve the rest in the refrigerator.

Peel the ginger knob and cut into small pieces. Set aside.

Now, combine beets, carrot, avocado, and ginger in a juicer. Process until well juiced and transfer to a serving glass. Stir in the and water and refrigerate for 5-10 minutes before serving.

Enjoy!

Nutrition information per serving: Kcal: 265, Protein: 5.9g, Carbs: 33.4g, Fats: 21.8g

33.   Cantaloupe Orange Juice

Ingredients:

1 cup cantaloupe, chopped

1 large orange, peeled

1 whole plum, chopped

1 cup fresh mint, torn

¼ tsp ginger, ground

Preparation:

Cut the cantaloupe in half. Scoop out the seeds and flesh. Cut and peel one large wedge. Chop into chunks and fill the measuring cup. Reserve the rest of the cantaloupe in a refrigerator.

Peel the orange and divide into wedges. Cut each wedge in half and set aside.

Wash the plum and cut in half. Remove the pit and chop into small pieces. Set aside.

Rinse the mint thoroughly under cold running water. Torn into small pieces and set aside.

Now, combine cantaloupe, orange, plum, and mint in a juicer and process until juiced. Transfer to a serving glass and stir in the ginger.

Add some ice and serve immediately.

Enjoy!

Nutrition information per serving: Kcal: 151, Protein: 4.4g, Carbs: 45.6g, Fats: 0.9g

34.   Apple Strawberry Juice

Ingredients:

1 cup blackberries

1 medium-sized Honeycrisp apple, cored and chopped

1 cup strawberries, chopped

1 large pear, chopped

¼ tsp cinnamon, ground

1 oz water

Preparation:

Wash the apple and cut lengthwise in half. Remove the core and chop into bite-sized pieces. Set aside.

Rinse strawberries and remove the stems. Cut into small pieces and fill the measuring cup. Reserve the rest in the refrigerator.

Wash the blackberries using a colander. Drain and set aside.

Wash the pear and cut in half. Remove the core and cut into small pieces. Set aside.

Now, combine apple, strawberries, blackberries, and pear in a juicer and process until well juiced. Transfer to a serving glass and stir in the cinnamon.

Refrigerate for 10 minutes before serving.

Enjoy!

Nutrition information per serving: Kcal: 246, Protein: 4.2g, Carbs: 82.1g, Fats: 1.7g

35.   Pomegranate Lemon Juice

Ingredients:

1 cup pomegranate seeds

1 whole lemon, peeled

1 cup fresh spinach, torn

2 oz water

Preparation:

Cut the top of the pomegranate fruit using a sharp paring knife. Slice down to each of the white membranes inside of the fruit. Pop the seeds into a measuring cup and set aside.

Peel the lemon and cut lengthwise in half. Set aside.

Rinse the spinach thoroughly under cold running water. Drain and torn into small pieces. Set aside.

Now, combine pomegranate seeds, spinach, and lemon in a juicer. Process until well juiced.

Transfer to a serving glass and stir in the water. Add some ice and serve immediately.

Enjoy!

Nutrition information per serving: Kcal: 195, Protein: 10.2g, Carbs: 56.1g, Fats: 2.1g

36.   Apple Guava Juice

Ingredients:

1 small Granny Smith's apple, cored and chopped

1 whole guava, chunked

1 cup strawberries, chopped

1 whole lemon, peeled and halved

¼ tsp cinnamon, ground

2 oz water

Preparation:

Wash the apple and cut lengthwise in half. Remove the core and cut into bite-sized pieces. Set aside.

Peel the guava and cut in half. Scoop out the seeds and wash it. Cut into small chunks and set aside.

Wash the strawberries and remove the stems. Cut into small pieces and fill the measuring cup. Reserve the rest in the refrigerator. Set aside.

Peel the lemon and cut lengthwise in half. Set aside.

Now, combine apple, guava, strawberries, and lemon in a juicer and process until juiced. Transfer to a serving glass and stir in the cinnamon and water.

Refrigerate for 5 minutes before serving.

Enjoy!

Nutrition information per serving: Kcal: 136, Protein: 3.6g, Carbs: 43.9g, Fats: 1.3g

37.   Banana Blueberry Juice

Ingredients:

1 large banana, peeled

1 cup blueberries

1 cup cherries, pitted

1 whole lemon, peeled

1 small Fuji apple, cored

¼ tsp cinnamon powder

Preparation:

Peel the banana and cut into small chunks. Set aside.

Rinse the blueberries using a large colander. Drain and set aside.

Wash the cherries and cut in half. Remove the pits and stems. Set aside.

Peel the lemon and cut lengthwise in half. Set aside.

Wash the apple and cut lengthwise in half. Remove the core and cut into small pieces. Set aside.

Now, combine banana, blueberries, cherries, lemon, and apple in a juicer and process until juiced. Transfer to a serving glass and stir in the cinnamon.

Add some ice and serve immediately.

Nutrition information per serving: Kcal: 340, Protein: 5.5g, Carbs: 102g, Fats: 1.7g

38. Apricot Banana Juice

Ingredients:

3 whole apricots, chopped

1 large banana, chunked

2 whole kiwis, peeled and halved

1 medium-sized Honeycrisp apple, cored and chopped

Preparation:

Wash the apricots and cut in half. Remove the pits and cut into small pieces. Set aside.

Peel the banana and cut into small chunks. Set aside.

Peel the kiwi and cut lengthwise in half. Set aside.

Wash the apple and cut lengthwise in half. Remove the core and cut into bite-sized pieces. Set aside.

Now, combine apricots, banana, kiwi, and apple in a juicer and process until juiced. Transfer to a serving glass and add some ice.

Serve immediately.

Nutrition information per serving: Kcal: 313, Protein: 5.4g, Carbs: 91g, Fats: 1.9g

39. Pineapple Lime Juice

Ingredients:

1 cup pineapple, chunked

1 whole lime, peeled

1 cup blackberries

1 large banana, sliced

2 oz water

Preparation:

Using a sharp paring knife, cut the top of the pineapple. Gently remove all hard skin and slice it into thin slices. Fill the measuring cup and reserve the rest for later.

Peel the lime and cut lengthwise in half. Set aside.

Place the blackberries in a small colander and wash under cold running water. Slightly drain and set aside.

Peel the banana and cut into thin slices. Set aside.

Now, combine pineapple, lime, blackberries, and banana in a juicer. Process until well juiced. Transfer to a serving glass and add some ice before serving.

Enjoy!

Nutrition information per serving: Kcal: 222, Protein: 4.5g, Carbs: 70.2g, Fats: 1.4g

40.   Asparagus Orange Juice

Ingredients:

1 cup asparagus, trimmed

3 medium-sized blood oranges, peeled and wedged

1 large Fuji apple, cored

¼ tsp ginger, ground

2 oz water

Preparation:

Rinse the asparagus thoroughly under cold running water using a colander. Trim off the woody ends. Cut into small pieces and set aside.

Peel the oranges and divide into wedges. Set aside.

Wash the apple and remove the core. Cut into bite-sized pieces and set aside.

Now, combine asparagus, oranges, and apple in a juicer and process until juiced. Transfer to serving glasses and stir in the ginger and water.

Refrigerate for 10 minutes before serving.

Nutrition information per serving: Kcal: 316, Protein: 9.1g, Carbs: 98.1g, Fats: 1.2g

41.   Broccoli Lemon Juice

Ingredients:

1 cup broccoli, chopped

1 whole lemon, peeled

1 large cucumber, sliced

1 cup avocado, chopped

1 large lime, peeled

1 oz water

Preparation:

Rinse the broccoli under running water. Chop into small pieces and fill the measuring cup. Set aside.

Peel the lemon and lime. Cut lengthwise in half. Set aside.

Peel the cucumber and cut in thick slices. Set aside.

Peel the avocado and cut in half. Remove the pit and cut into chunks. Set aside.

Now, combine broccoli, lemon, cucumber, avocado, and lime in a juicer. Process until juiced. Transfer to serving glasses and stir in the water.

Add some ice and serve immediately.

Nutritional information per serving: Kcal: 281, Protein: 8.3g, Carbs: 38.8g, Fats: 22.8g

42. Orange Cucumber Juice

Ingredients:

2 large oranges, peeled

1 large cucumber, peeled

1 cup broccoli, chopped

1 large carrot, sliced

1 oz water

Preparation:

Peel the oranges and divide into wedges. Set aside.

Wash the cucumber and cut into thin slices. Set aside.

Wash the broccoli and trim off the outer leaves. Cut into small pieces and fill the measuring cup. Reserve the rest in the refrigerator.

Now, combine oranges, cucumber, broccoli, and carrot in a juicer and process until juiced.

Transfer to a serving glass and stir in the water.

Add few ice cubes and serve immediately!

Nutritional information per serving: Kcal: 68, Protein: 2.3g, Carbs: 19.7g, Fats: 0.1g

43.   Apple Lemon Juice

Ingredients:

1 large Granny Smith's apple, cored

1 whole lemon, peeled

3 medium-sized celery stalks, chopped

½ cup freh cilantro, chopped

¼ tsp ginger powder

1 tsp maple syrup

Preparation:

Wash the apple and cut in half. Remove the core and cut into small pieces. Set aside.

Peel the lemon and cut lengthwise in half. Set aside.

Rinse the celery and chop into small pieces. Set aside.

Now, combine apple, lemon, celery, and cilantro in a juicer. Process until juiced. Transfer to serving glasses and stir in the ginger and maple syrup.

Add few ice cubes and serve immediately.

Nutritional information per serving: Kcal: 153, Protein: 2.3g, Carbs: 38.4g, Fats: 0.2g

44. Banana Pomegranate Juice

Ingredients:

1 large banana, chunked

1 cup pomegranate seeds

1 medium-sized Honeycrisp apple, cored

1 tbsp agave nectar

1 oz water

Preparation:

Peel the banana and cut into small chunks. Set aside.

Cut the top of the pomegranate fruit using a sharp paring knife. Slice down to each of the white membranes inside of the fruit. Pop the seeds into a measuring cup and set aside.

Wash the apple and cut lengthwise in half. Remove the core and cut into bite-sized pieces. Set aside.

Now, combine banana, pomegranate seeds, and apple in a juicer. Process until juiced. Transfer to a serving glass and stir in the agave nectar and water.

Serve cold.

Nutrition information per serving: Kcal: 243, Protein: 3.6g, Carbs: 70.1g, Fats: 1.8g

45.   Artichoke Cherry Juice

Ingredients:

1 cup artichokes, chopped

1 cup fresh cherries, pitted

1 whole lemon, peeled

1 medium-sized Fuji apple, cored

¼ tsp cinnamon, ground

Preparation:

Rinse the artichoke and trim off the outer, hard leaves. Cut into bite-sized pieces and fill the measuring cup. Reserve the rest in the refrigerator.

Rinse the cherries under running water using a colander. Cut each in half and remove the pits. Set aside.

Peel the lemon and cut lengthwise in half. Set aside.

Wash the apple and cut lengthwise in half. Remove the core and cut into bite-sized pieces. Set aside.

Now, combine artichoke, cherries, lemon, and apple in a juicer and process until juiced. Transfer to a serving glass and stir in the cinnamon.

Refrigerate for 10 minutes before serving.

Nutrition information per serving: Kcal: 205, Protein: 7.2g, Carbs: 66.2g, Fats: 0.9g

46.   Carrot Celery Juice

Ingredients:

1 medium-sized carrot, sliced

1 cup celery, chopped

1 small Roma tomato, chopped

1 cup fresh spinach, torn

¼ tsp salt

¼ tsp balsamic vinegar

Preparation:

Wash and peel the carrot. Cut into thin slices and set aside.

Wash the celery and chop into small pieces. Set aside.

Wash the tomato and place in a small bowl. Cut into bite-sized pieces. Make sure to reserve the tomato juice while cutting. Set aside.

Wash the spinach thoroughly under cold running water. Torn into small pieces and set aside.

Now, combine carrot, celery, tomato, and spinach in a juicer. Process until juiced. Transfer to a serving glass and stir in the salt, vinegar, and reserved tomato juice.

Refrigerate for 20 minutes before serving.

Nutrition information per serving: Kcal: 72, Protein: 8.4g, Carbs: 21.2g, Fats: 1.4g

47.   Apple Watermelon Juice

Ingredients:

1 medium-sized Granny Smith's apple, cored and chopped

1 cup watermelon, cubed

1 large peach, pitted and chopped

1 banana, peeled and sliced

¼ tsp cinnamon, ground

Preparation:

Wash the apple and cut in half. Remove the core and cut into bite-sized pieces. Set aside.

Cut the watermelon in half. Cut one large wedge and wrap the rest in a plastic foil and refrigerate. Peel the slice and cut into small cubes. Remove the pits and fill the measuring cup. Set aside.

Wash the peach and cut lengthwise in half. Remove the pit and chop into bite-sized pieces. Set aside.

Peel the banana and cut into thin slices. Set aside.

Now, combine watermelon, peach, apple, and banana in a juicer and process until juiced. Transfer to a serving glass and stir in the cinnamon.

Add some ice and serve immediately!

Nutrition information per serving: Kcal: 260, Protein: 4.4g, Carbs: 73.9g, Fats: 1.3g

48.   Grape Spinach Juice

Ingredients:

1 cup black grapes

1 cup fresh spinach, torn

1 cup broccoli, chopped

1 small Granny Smith's apple, cored

1 tbsp fresh mint, finely chopped

Preparation:

Rinse the grapes under running water and remove the stems. Set aside.

Using a large colander, rinse the broccoli and spinach under cold running water. Drain and torn the spinach in small pieces. Trim off the outer leaves of the broccoli and cut into small pieces. Fill the measuring cups and set aside.

Wash the apple and cut lengthwise in half. Remove the core and cut into bite-sized pieces. Set aside.

Now, combine grapes, spinach, broccoli, and apple in a juicer and process until well juiced. Transfer to a serving glass and sprinkle with some fresh mint.

Refrigerate for 10 minutes before serving.

Nutrition information per serving: Kcal: 176, Protein: 9.8g, Carbs: 49.5g, Fats:1.7g

49.   Avocado Lettuce Juice

Ingredients:

1 cup avocado, chunked

1 cup Iceberg lettuce, chopped

1 large carrot, chopped

1 cup collard greens, torn

1 cucumber, sliced

¼ tsp ginger, ground

Preparation:

Peel the avocado and cut lengthwise in half. Remove the pit and cut into small chunks. Fill the measuring cup and reserve the rest in the refrigerator.

Wash and peel the carrot. Cut into thin slices and set aside.

Place lettuce and collard greens in a large colander. Rinse well thoroughly under cold running water. Drain and chop into small pieces. Set aside.

Wash the cucumber and cut into thin slices. Fill the measuring cup and reserve the rest for later. Set aside.

Now, combine avocado, lettuce, carrot, collard greens, and cucumber in a juicer and process until juiced. Transfer to a serving glass and stir in the ginger.

Refrigerate for 5 minutes before serving.

Nutrition information per serving: Kcal: 271, Protein: 7.3g, Carbs: 34.1g, Fats: 22.8g

ADDITIONAL TITLES FROM THIS AUTHOR

70 Effective Meal Recipes to Prevent and Solve Being Overweight: Burn Fat Fast by Using Proper Dieting and Smart Nutrition

By Joe Correa CSN

48 Acne Solving Meal Recipes: The Fast and Natural Path to Fixing Your Acne Problems in Less Than 10 Days!

By Joe Correa CSN

41 Alzheimer's Preventing Meal Recipes: Reduce or Eliminate Your Alzheimer's Condition in 30 Days or Less!

By Joe Correa CSN

70 Effective Breast Cancer Meal Recipes: Prevent and Fight Breast Cancer with Smart Nutrition and Powerful Foods

By Joe Correa CSN

www.ingramcontent.com/pod-product-compliance
Lightning Source LLC
Chambersburg PA
CBHW030257030426
42336CB00009B/422